How to Lose Man Boobs Fast and Naturally

I0426623

Get Rid of Man Boobs Once and for All

Kenneth L.David

Copyright

© 2013 by Kenneth L.David

ISBN: 978-1-304-27981-1

All rights reserved. No part of this book may be reproduced, copied, stored, or transmitted in any form or by any means, electronic, photographic, or mechanical, including photocopying, recording, or in any information storage and retrieval systems, without prior written permission of the author, except where permitted by copyright law.

This information is not presented by a medical practitioner and is for educational and informational purposes only. The content is not intended to be a substitute for professional medical advice, diagnosis, or treatment. Always seek the advice of your physician or other qualified health provider with any questions you may have regarding a medical condition. Never disregard professional medical advice or delay in seeking it because of something you have read.

Contents

Introduction

Man boobs are a source of embarrassment for men who have them. When you have man boobs or a flabby chest, you tend to leave your shirt on while at the beach, while at the pool, while mowing the lawn or while doing anything really, even though it might be hot outside.

You can be toned and fit otherwise but man boobs tend to linger and they are humiliating. There are a ton of products on the market that are all designed to help get rid of man boobs, but truth be told, none of them work.

Man boobs can be something that you are born with and that do not show up until later on in your life or it can be something that happens, as you get older for some reason, often due to obesity, hormonal imbalances, or illness.

Because hormone imbalance is a common factor, no amount of exercise, either aerobic or target chest weight training will help.

It will boost your overall health, but not get rid of your man boobs, which is a very frustrating thing to have happen.

If you have man boobs, you might feel that you are stuck with them, or that you need to take drastic measures and get surgery, which is a very costly problem, and if a hormone imbalance is the cause of your man boobs, then it will only be a temporary fix, or you can work to reverse the process.

Our book will educate you on the many reasons that you might have man boobs and how to reverse the problem.

Once you know more about why you have man boobs, it is easier to begin working on reversing the process, shedding your man boobs, and giving yourself a chest that you can be proud of once again.

We will focus on how to limit your exposure to the environment factors that contribute to your man boobs.

Yes, your environment has a great deal to do with your man boobs and why they are so stubborn about going away.

We will go over what foods to avoid and what foods to eat to help put your hormones back into balance.

Lastly, we will go over exercises that are natural testosterone boosting exercises. However, you can get rid of your man boobs and you can do so safely, without buying into gimmicks.

Welcome to the beginning of having a chest that you can be proud of!

What are Man Boobs?

There are numerous reasons why a man can develop what looks like breast. Gynaecomastia is the medical terminology for having developed male breasts.

Turcios Disease is the terminology for man boobs themselves and they can be present from birth, develop at puberty or when the male is an adult, there is no clear-cut trigger for what causes them to suddenly grow.

One of the reasons for having man boobs is because the mammary glands develop to an abnormally large size, resulting in gynaecomastia, or man boobs.

In some extreme cases, these abnormally large mammary glands actually end up producing milk. So why do the mammary glands develop abnormally in some men, and not in others?

There is no single explanation as to why this happens to some men, and not to others. As with anything, there are many theories out there and for a male who has this condition; it can be any one of them, or a combination of several reasons.

What is known is that the men who have the condition tend to have lower self-esteem and lack confidence.

The biggest culprit for causing man boobs is a balance in your hormones.

Men and women store fat in different places, men often store fat in their bellies, hence the male "beer belly" however, if a male has a hormone imbalance, then they tend store fat equally between their chest and their belly.

When it comes to hormones, people tend to think that men have only testosterone in their bodies and women have only estrogen and that would be incorrect.

Men and women have both hormones in their system, only women have more estrogen and men have more testosterone and when they have more estrogen or less testosterone than they should, it is a hormonal imbalance and developing man boobs is a result of that.

Testosterone is the hormone that causes the development of the male characteristics such as muscle mass, body hair, facial hair, reproductive system development, and the deep voice.

However, in the body, some testosterone is converted to estrogen, because men need some estrogen as well, so trying to balance the hormones by taking testosterone will not work because the body will just convert some to estrogen and the imbalance will continue.

Estrogen is the hormone that causes the female characteristics to grow in women, such as breasts, body hair, and regulates their reproductive cycle.

If a man has more estrogen in his system than normal, he will experience erectile dysfunction, weight gain, a decrease in muscle mass and development of breasts, or man boobs.

If you suddenly develop man boobs, when it is not a problem that you have had before, you should see a doctor to rule out any medical conditions that could be causing a hormone imbalance.

Kidney and liver problems are a common reason for your body to have an imbalance so if you suddenly get man boobs where you have not had them before please, see a doctor right away.

You should also get your prostrate checked because if your testosterone level decreases, man boobs is a result. Men do get breast cancer, another cause of the increase in the breast tissue mass, and things like alcoholism and cirrhosis can also cause man boobs.

Does being overweight contribute to having man boobs? Yes, being overweight is a significant reason for having man boobs.

When you are overweight, you carry extra fat in your body. The extra fat will settle in your belly and your breasts, making the condition that much more noticeable.

If you are obese, your man boobs are likely just due to your weight, however, being overweight is in itself a factor in causing the hormone imbalance in the first place so it is always a good idea to work to get to a healthy weight, not only to shed your man boobs, but for your overall health in the first place.

Steroid use is another factor. Synthetic steroids are a popular choice for body builders because it helps to build muscle mass and reduce fat.

Steroids enter the body and the body thinks that the steroids are extra testosterone and treats them as such and remember how we said that it would convert to estrogen, which is exactly what will happen.

Steroids given medically, such as for treating cancer, AIDS, to initiate puberty, stimulate bone growth and appetite will also cause male breasts to form.

Some medication actually contains hormones and so males taking these medicines will end up developing man boobs because of the hormones that they are putting into their body.

They may not even realize that this will be a side effect of the medication.

Medicines that can disrupt the hormone balance to cause man boobs include Omeprazole, Cimetidine, Spironolactone, Imatinib mesylate and some antipsychotics, tricyclic antidepressants, ulcer medication, some chemotherapy drugs, and some chemotherapy medication.

Many of the drugs used to treat prostate cancer, such as cyproterone and flutamide, will cause man boobs, so if you are currently being treated for that, the condition is a side effect of the treatment and talk to your doctor about it.

If you are in constant contact with a female who is wearing a progesterone patch, the progesterone in the patch can actually transfer to you, through skin contact, which can lower your testosterone levels.

Environmental and Other Causes

Hormones in the environment can also affect men. The things that we encounter during our day and even the things that we put into our bodies can actually enhance the hormone imbalance.

So what else can cause a hormone imbalance in men?

Environment toxins are a significant culprit for causing hormone imbalances in men and women.

Many of the everyday products that we encounter contain chemicals that are toxic and can disrupt our hormone production; endocrine disruptors is the term for these.

These chemicals are prevalent in plastics, and although we do not eat plastic, we are in constant contact with it, and indeed, we wrap much of our food in plastic.

Pesticides and herbicides are also high with endocrine disruptors, and these are found in our produce and in any grain based food that is not labeled as organic; which is why eating organic is a smart choice.

Our air and water supply has these toxins as well and cleaning products are another big cause of endocrine disrupters.

Xenoestrogens are one of the types of endocrine disruptors and the main one that is the cause of man boobs.

Xenoestrogens enter our bodies and are similar enough to our natural hormones, that our body gets confused and disrupts our normal hormone production. Plastics, fungicides, herbicides, and pesticides all contain xenoestrogens.

When they enter your body, these xenoestrogens can impact your metabolic system, immune system, nervous system, endocrine system, and your reproductive system.

They are hard to get rid of as well because not only can they not be broken down and excreted by our bodies but they actually stay in our fat cells and other tissues so that once they are in our bodies, they tend to stay there, compounding the hormone imbalance.

So how do you avoid these environment toxins?

First of all, the best way is to promote green living, such as recycling and buying products made from recycling materials; it may not help your problem, but it will help reduce the toxins in the environment.

If you use pesticides or herbicides, switch to all natural ways products to solve the problem. You can get rid of bugs and weeds without using toxins.

Use all natural cleaning products; this will eliminate a lot of your environmental exposure. Even things that seem harmless, like air freshener, contain endocrine disruptors.

Your diet affects your hormones, and we will go into this in more detail in later chapters, but diets that are high in white flour, sugar, caffeine, and refined carbohydrates will contribute to the hormonal imbalance and the development of man boobs.

A diet in which those foods are heavily consumed means that you are eating things with little or no nutritional value, and proper nutrition is vital to shedding your man boobs.

Many of the meats that we buy and dairy products have hormones in them, because the animals are given hormones to help them grow bigger.

Not just meat has hormones, but dairy as well, products liked yogurt, cottage cheese, milk, and eggs.

Look for hormone free brands and perhaps buy locally, where the chance of hormones being in your food is less. Foods that are antibiotic and hormone free will be labeled as such.

If you have an imbalance in your neurotransmitters, it can also cause an imbalance in your hormones.

Avoid things that will cause a disruption in your neurotransmitters such as, drugs, alcohol, nicotine, lack of proper protein and refined sugar.

Stress causes your endocrine system to go into overdrive and this will cause a deficiency in neurotransmitters, causing a hormone imbalance.

If you are experiencing a significant amount of stress, you need to find ways to relax such as exercise, deep breathing relaxation techniques, and meditation.

Chronic stress is a huge factor in hormone imbalances and the longer you allow your body to run in stress mode, the worse the problem will become.

There are great many things that can create a hormonal imbalance, and that is where this book comes in handy, because that is the problem that we can address, that along with being at a healthy weight, will help you finally loose the man boobs.

The Importance of Hydration

Many of us grew up being told to drink at least eight glasses of water a day and many of us let that advice go in one ear and out the other.

However, in this case, your mom was right; you really need to drink at least eight glasses of water a day.

We tend to think that as long as we are drinking fluids that we are getting enough water. Sodas, iced teas, coffee, tea, even many of the juices that we can buy are full of water and so we get complacent and we think that well, it contains water so that's good enough!

That thinking is incorrect and as a result, the majority of the population is dehydrated and they do not even realize it. Between 50% to 65% of the general population is dehydrated on any given day.

When you are dehydrated, you have trouble concentrating, you get headaches and you feel tired; but dehydration is also a factor in regulating hormone production and so when you are dehydrated, your hormones can become imbalanced.

Other fluids, even sports drinks and fitness waters, are not equal substitutions for water. The only liquid that properly rehydrates the human body is water.

If you drink alcohol, soda or fruit juices you are only contributing to your own dehydration because the acidic nature of those drinks only causes you to become further dehydrated.

They might taste good when you are thirsty, but drinking soda, alcohol, and commercially bottled fruit juices will quench your thirst but make the dehydration worse, which in turns compounds the hormonal imbalance.

We will go further into how an alkaline diet can improve the hormonal imbalance, but regular water itself, due to being treated and even polluted, is only slightly alkaline.

Increasing your intake of alkaline foods is a great way to help lose your man boobs, but since we talking about hydration right now, here is a little tip that falls into both categories, add some lemon juice to your water!

A lot of people avoid drinking water because they do not like the taste. They find water bland, which is why they tend to drink unhealthy choices, often laden with preservatives and chemicals, none of which is healthy to ingest.

If you are one of the ones that simply do not like the taste of water, adding lemon juice to your water is a great way to give your water a splash of flavor, with a very valuable side effect, one that can actually help to reverse the growth of man boobs.

We advised you to stay away from juices, sodas and alcohol because the acidic nature of those can make you even more dehydrated but when it comes to increasing the alkalinity in your body, that is the right sort of acid.

Lemon is highly alkaline when processed by the body and so by adding lemon to your water you are not only improving the flavor of the water, but helping to shed the man boobs.

You should be drinking at least eight glasses of water a day, at a minimum. When you consider how much you actually drink during the day, it is easy to get to eight glasses of water because you just have to substitute your colas, juices, coffees, energy drinks, and other beverages with water.

If you are at a restaurant, request water and a few lemon slices, that way you can squeeze some lemon into your water and still get a tasty, refreshing, and very beneficial drink.

Once you get into the habit of drinking enough water you will find it easier to keep it up, and you will start to feel much better! You will probably wonder why you have not done this before.

Filtered water is the best type of water to drink. You can keep a supply of cut lemon wedges in your refrigerator so that when you get water, it is easy to squeeze lemon into it.

You can even keep a pitcher of filtered water in the refrigerator with lemon already in it, so that all you need to do is pour when you are home, and needing a drink.

When at work, you can bring your lemon infused water with you, bring enough to get you through the day and keep it in the office refrigerator. As an alternative, you can bring a jug of water with you.

Here is where it gets tricky. Most plastic has BPA chemicals in them, chemicals that leech into the water; these are the chemicals that we were talking about in the prior chapter, the chemicals that cause hormone imbalance.

This is why we say to use filtered water, do not buy bottled water, unless it is stamped as being filtered water in a bottle then contains no BPA plastics.

Thanks to the nation's growing concern over health issues and to protect the environment, it is easier to find products that are made from recycled plastic already or that are made without the use of BPAs.

Drinking water will also help to flush toxins and waste products out of your body, which will help your body shed some of the products and toxins that are lingering, contributing to the imbalance of hormones.

We have been talking about avoiding juices. At this point, we need to clarify that the juices that we are recommending are commercially produced and bottled juices that you buy in the store.

Fresh apple juice and orange juice that you make yourself, or buy that are 100% juice and not from concentrate are excellent to drink, but you still need to drink eight glasses of water a day.

You just have to be diligent when it comes to reading labels and if the orange or apple juice is not 100% juice, do not buy it. Consider investing in a juicer and making your own fresh and healthy juice at home.

Green tea is a good tea to drink for losing weight, and it contains caffeine so you will not have to endure caffeine withdrawal that would happen if you went cold turkey on no caffeine.

Substitute green tea for your morning coffee and you can make iced tea with green tea and add lemon to it. Fennel seed tea and oolong tea are both teas that are recommended for people who are trying to lose weight.

Since obesity contributes to man boobs, when you lose the fat, the man boobs will also be reduced.

If you like your tea sweetened, avoid sugar, and avoid sugar substitutes. Honey is an excellent way to sweeten your tea; it is diet friendly and a natural substance, which is always a better choice.

Another drink that is good is one that most people might wrinkle up their nose at, but it tastes much better than it looks, we promise! That drink is to juice dark leafy vegetables, such as kale, because they are also highly alkaline. You can juice them yourself at home or you can buy them from health food stores or even in the grocery section, Naked Juice is one such brand that you can buy.

As you can see, there are more options for staying hydrated than just water, so you are not looking at a diet devoid of flavorful drinks.

When you drink tea or juice, it does not count as a glass of water, so you still need to drink eight full glasses a day, preferable with lemon in it.

Although it may take your body a few days to adjust to the extra fluid, you will begin to feel better and look better.

Your entire system will benefit from drinking enough water; it will do more than just help to balance your hormones.

Breathing Right

It may seem silly that you can help reduce man boobs by simply breathing. However, it really can be a factor!

When your body becomes too acidic, it can cause the imbalance that helps encourage the development of man boobs.

Breathing techniques have been used historically in every culture as a way to healing. It is perhaps one of the most enduring ancient healing methods because it works.

Why else would nearly every culture develop a healing method that includes focusing on breathing? Breathing matters!

Through controlled breathing, you can control a lot about your body.

Controlled breathing can help with stress, and remember how stress is a contributing factor to man boobs; well-controlled breathing is one way to force your body into a calmer zone.

Controlled breathing can also lower blood pressure, and energize you, because when you do deep breathing, you are increasing the oxygen levels in your blood.

We tend to breathe shallow, using our lungs, and so we get oxygen, but not enough oxygen.

By breathing deeply, using your abdomen, you can increase your oxygen, which will help you feel better and extra oxygen into your bloodstream will have other benefits.

We have talked a little about how having a higher level on alkaline in your body can help to reverse the hormonal damage, and while having a high acid level is not ideal conditions for health, increasing the alkalinity in your system does have benefits, one of which is reducing man boobs.

When you use breathing techniques to cleanse and detoxify your body by improving your oxygen intake, it prepares your body to be better equipped to handle more alkalinity.

The very act of breathing increases the alkalinity of our blood. As we exhale carbon dioxide, our blood becomes alkalinized.

The goal is to not bounce back and forth from alkalinized state and a non-alkalinized state, but to try to keep a steady alkaline state.

Ragged breathing, rapid breathing, and shallow breathing all means that we are taking in inconsistent oxygen levels and can lead to an inconsistent alkaline level and that is why deep breathing is so important.

Breathing exercises are designed to make sure that you are exchanging equal amounts of oxygen and carbon dioxide; which means that you keep your breathing steady and measured.

The more oxygen that you have in your body, the easier it will be for your body to absorb alkaline foods.

As you eat things that are alkaline, having enough oxygen in your body is vital to having your body be able to properly process the alkaline foods and therefore, reducing your man boobs.

There are a number of ways that you can learn to breathe better, yoga classes or meditation sessions nearly always include breathing techniques, like we said, deep breathing is used all over the world for a variety of reasons, the benefits of it are well documented.

How exactly do you do a deep breathing exercise?

This is only one example, because there are a variety of them out there, no one way is better than the rest, as long as you breathing deep and slow you will be receiving the benefits of the exercise.

The trick to deep breathing is to breathe from deep in your belly; your stomach should expand, not your chest.

When you inhale from the abdomen, you get more air because the lower section of your lungs can contain more air, and inhaling through your abdomen fills your lungs starting from the lower sections first.

When you breathe with your chest, you are only filling up the top part of your lungs.

When you breathe, you need to inhale deeply and exhale fully because shallow exhales never expel all of the toxins that you need to; you need to fully expel all of the air in your lungs to detoxify your body and ensure that your breathing is giving you the maximum benefit.

Take a deep breath in, counting to three as you inhale to ensure that you are breathing deeply enough.

Imagine as you inhale that the air is entering your body and filling your lungs from the bottom up, count to three while you inhale and then hold the air in your lungs for four seconds, allowing the oxygen to enter your body, and then slowly exhale, to a count of four as well.

Repeat this around five times.

This is a very good breathing exercise to do when you feel stressed or anxious; it will instantly calm you down.

Supplements

Now, we said that you could lose your man boobs without buying gimmicks or products that do not work.

With that being said, there are plenty of supplements that you can take, that will help you reduce your man boobs, and that are all natural.

Avoid products that say that they will boost your testosterone. At present, the only way to boost testosterone will be to have it done though prescription medication.

There is a wealth of products out there promising to increase your testosterone to correct the imbalance and therefore, getting rid of your man boobs.

Some supplements might have a slight effect on your testosterone, but it will not actually increase it to any great degree.

Those products are not to be trusted and will either be a waste of money, or actually harmful to you. If a pill would increase your testosterone levels, the same people who abuse steroids would abuse the supplements.

The very fact that these supplements that claim to increase testosterone are allowed on the shelves proves that they do not work, if they did, they would be considered a banned substance, just like steroids.

Therefore, that is just a warning about products to avoid. Avoid things that are telling you that they will magically work.

We are not saying that there are things that you can take that will make your man boobs go away overnight, but what we are saying is that there are supplements that you can take that will help reduce them over time.

The supplements that we are going talk about are all natural supplements, things that will have only positive changes to your health and that will help you reduce your man boobs, either by helping to bring your hormones back into balance naturally, or to help increase the alkalinity of your body, which has the same result.

The mineral Zinc is vital to helping your body produce testosterone and our body gets rid of zinc easily, meaning that it is very easy to become zinc deficient, which can affect how much testosterone that we have in our body.

Zinc does not create an increase in testosterone, but it helps our bodies produce it, which is why it is vital.

As we sweat, we sweat out zinc, so anything that we do that produces sweat, such as sex, exercise, even mowing the lawn, causes us to lose zinc.

You should take one zinc supplement at night, with a full glass of water, right before you go to bed. Take it on an empty stomach for best results.

You can eat zinc rich foods as well, but taking a supplement ensures that you have enough in your system; some foods that include zinc are oysters, wheat germ, lean roast beef, roasted pumpkin seeds, liver, cocoa and dark chocolate, mutton, peanuts and crab.

We already mentioned that stress can cause a hormone imbalance, the reason it does that is because stress releases cortisol, which hinders the body's production of DHEA, which, like zinc, is necessary for producing testosterone in our bodies. DHEA is available as a supplement and taking at least 25mg a day will help counter the effects of cortisol.

If you are prone to stress and are living with chronic stress, DHEA is a supplement that you should be taking because it will help to negate and actually reverse the damage that cortisol has done to your body.

DHEA is legal to buy through health stores and nutrition shops in the United States; however, if you are an athlete, you should not take DHEA because the use of it is banned in athletic competitions.

Aloe vera juice is another way to increase your alkalinity. You can buy aloe vera juice at health food stores, all natural food stores, and nutrition stores.

When you have too much acid in your system you end up with irritation and inflammation, aloe vera is a natural way to get rid of that inflammation. When you control the inflammation, it will help improve the balance in your body between acidity and alkaline conditions.

When you think of hydrogen peroxide, you think of wound cleansing, because that is traditionally what it has been used for.

However, hydrogen peroxide is another way that you can increase your body's alkalinity. **Do not drink or ingest hydrogen peroxide that you buy in the store!**

Do not take hydrogen peroxide that you buy in the store and try to drink it or to add it to your beverages – **doing so will make you ill and can cause bodily harm.**

Health food stores sell supplements that are designed to be mixed with water and ingested, the hydrogen peroxide in bottles that you find in regular stores is NOT safe to use.

Only purchase hydrogen peroxide supplements from well-known health food and nutrition stores and use only as directed.

Mineral salts are another way that you can increase the alkalinity of your body.

You need to have enough potassium, magnesium, iron, manganese, and calcium in your diet to help increase your alkalinity, and often if you take them in a supplement, they will also contain amino acids and digestive enzymes to help you absorb them better.

Taking supplements does no good if they pass through your system without being absorbed.

Calcium is especially important because when your body is too acidic, your body tries to correct that by pulling calcium from your bones to restore a balance and that can lead to bone loss, brittle bones, and osteoporosis.

You can find supplements that contain all or most of these mineral salts to avoid having to take them all individually, but calcium is perhaps the most important one, so make sure that you have a supplement that contains calcium as well, or take a separate supplement for calcium.

Omega oils are another very important supplement to have in your diet. Omega-3, Omega-6, and Omega-9 oils that are essential to keeping your endocrine system functioning like it is supposed to, especially your kidneys.

Flaxseed and fish are two great sources of omega oils and you can find both in the vitamin and supplement aisles of nearly any grocery store or drug store.

Vitamin D is vital to have in your body because without it, your body would not process calcium properly and vitamin D actually helps to elevate the levels of testosterone in your body.

You can take vitamin D as a supplement or you can spend an hour a day outside because with exposure to sunlight, our bodies actually will produce vitamin D!

Antioxidants are substances that work to prevent, hold off, or even reverse damage to our cells. Of course, because those environmental toxins end up in our bodies, we need to do our best to cleanse them out, to get them out of the stored fat cells and gone. Antioxidants are one such way.

One phrase that you will find associated with antioxidant supplements is the ORAC value. ORAC is the Oxygen Radical Absorption Capacity and since you want things to be absorbed better, the higher this number, the more effective the supplement.

Acai berry supplements have a high ORAC value and are a very good supplement to take to help get rid of your man boobs, they are full of antioxidants, and you will be feeling and looking better with regular use.

Gluthathione, goji berry juice, CoQ 10, Spirulina, alpha lipoic acid, beta carotene, vitamin E, garlic, green tea extract, grape seed extract, lycopene, and rooibos red tea are all examples of antioxidants that can be taken in supplement form that will help you get healthy, cleanse your body and help you get rid of your man boobs, once and for all.

Avoid These Foods

Although we will go over losing weight in more detail later on, we are going to use this section as a stepping-stone to our section on weight loss because no matter if you are overweight or not, eating certain foods will only make your man boobs more pronounced.

What you eat is important. We tend to just eat without giving much thought about what we are eating or how it will affect us.

In today's fast-paced lifestyle, everything is pre-packaged for convenience. Foods are ready to eat and we have to do very little to prepare them.

However, this grab and go way of eating is detrimental to our health. Not only does it contribute greatly to obesity, but also it can actually make your man boobs more pronounced, even if you are not over weight.

That is food for thought, is it not? What we eat can make a big difference in our health, but we do not stop to consider that when we are busy or hungry.

We see something that is ready to eat, tastes good and that take virtually no preparation. We can eat while driving, while at our desk, or while on the go, running errands or anything else.

These are not healthy choices and not only are they destroying your health, but they are accentuate your man boobs, because these foods contribute to the problem.

You will need to change your eating habits. We will go more into what you need to eat in later sections, just like we will go into some basic weight loss tips in later sections as well, but for now, we are going to concentrate on what you should NOT be eating.

Foods that need to come out of your diet or be limited in the quantity and frequency that you consume them.

First on the list are saturated fats. A diet high in saturated fats is a major contributing factor to heart disease, because it will clog your arteries.

High cholesterol levels are another health hazard caused by too many saturated fats in the diet, and high cholesterol can lead to heart disease and even cancer.

Saturated fats also contribute to obesity, and because men who have man boobs tend to have their extra weight settle in their chest and their stomachs, it will cause your man boobs to grow larger than they are.

If you want to reduce your man boobs, you need to change your eating habits to avoid these. Cheese, whole milk, butter, red meat, palm oil, coconut butter, and other dairy products all contain saturated fats.

Trans-fats are just as bad at saturated fats and worse yet, you cannot read a label to see if they contain trans-fats or not.

However, if you read a label and the product contains either partially hydrogenated or hydrogenated vegetable oil, it will be high in trans-fats and should be avoid. Foods that contain these are margarine, cakes, fried foods, frostings, and pies.

To reduce and get rid of your man boobs, sodium is something that needs to be reduced. Your sodium intake should be under 2,500mg a day.

Nearly all processed foods contain high amounts of sodium as do frozen foods and certain meats. Yes, those diet TV dinner might be low calorie but their sodium content is extremely high because everything is processed.

Lunchmeat, hot dogs, cheese, dried soup mixes, frozen dinners, heat and eat foods such as frozen burritos and pizzas, and pasta and potato box mixes are all high in sodium.

Snack foods that are high in refined sugar are also something that you need to avoid. Pastries, cookies, candies, brownies and other similar products are simply not healthy for you to eat.

Another reason to avoid the pre-packaged and ready to heat and eat meals is that they are packaged in and with plastic.

Plastic is a contributor to the whole issue of the hormone imbalance so it is just smart to avoid eating this as much as possible, because not only they are high in sodium, but also they increase your chances of continuing to have the BPA toxins leech into your food, contributing to the problem of having man boobs.

Limit your bread, pasta, and rice intake. These will only contribute to your weight gain, or make losing weight harder and you will have difficulty losing your man boobs.

Weight is a Factor

Simply stated, if you are overweight you will have man boobs. You do not have to be overweight to have a problem with man boobs, but being overweight compounds the problem.

The more fat that you have to store, the bigger your man boobs will be.

For overweight and obese men, sometimes all that they need to do to lose the man boobs is to lose weight, getting themselves down to a healthy weight.

If there is no excess fat in the body, there will be no excess fat to store in breasts. If you have man boobs and you are overweight, you need to make losing weight a priority if you want to lose your man boobs.

It is the first step to not only having a longer and healthier life, but the first step in shedding the man boobs that you want to get rid of.

The more weight you carry on you, the bigger your man boobs will be so managing your weight is the first step towards getting rid of your man boobs.

Before you rush out to buy a gym membership and buy a bunch of health food or purchase into a diet plan, there is one thing that you need to do first.

You need to decide that you want to lose weight and that you CAN lose weight.

Losing weight is not easy and it will be challenging. You need to get yourself mentally prepared, because you will be making big changes.

Think of all of the positive things that will happen once you start losing weight, not only will your man boobs start to reduce, but you will look better all around, feel better, have more energy and more self-esteem and confidence than ever before!

You can make plans all you want to lose weight, but until you actually take action, it is all talk. You need to take action and not just talk about it.

Why wait until tomorrow to start losing weight, making excuses for yourself will not help you get rid of the man boobs.

Taking action will help you get rid of them. Be decisive and take action, every day that you procrastinate is another day that your man boobs remain.

Start focusing on the positive outcomes that will come with losing weight, motivate yourself to do so and stick with it. So how can you motivate yourself?

One of the best ways to motivate yourself is to take a picture of yourself when you were thinner and put it where you can see it.

As a matter of fact, you should have several pictures of yourself looking as thin as you want to be, without man boobs for this idea.

If you have always had man boobs or have always been overweight, do not worry. Print out some pictures from online or cut them out from men's magazines of men with the body type that you want.

Tape one to the mirror in the bathroom, one to the refrigerator, one on your closet, and even put on where you eat your meals, such as on the table or a counter, and one on your pantry door.

Whenever you wander in for a snack, take a look at the picture and think, do you really need that snack?

Visual motivation is very good for keeping your motivated while you are working on losing weight.

Chart or track your progress so you can see that what you are doing is working. Nothing motivates like progress!

It might be slow going at first and there will always be times when your progress seems to stall but that is totally normal and to be expected.

When that happens, do not worry and just keep doing what you are doing and you will push through the plateau and will begin to see progress again. Weight yourself first thing in the morning weekly and write it down.

You should also measure your chest, waist and even your arms and thighs if you want and write it down. As you see the numbers start to go down you will know that you are doing good and it will serve as continued motivation!

Take a weekly photo of yourself and store it in a folder on your phone or computer. As you start to lose weight, you will be able to see your progression towards being thinner right before your eyes, another big motivator.

Find a weight loss buddy. Even if you do not have a friend who has man boobs, you doubtless have a friend who wants to lose weight.

With a weight loss buddy, the two of you can motivate each other, keep each other on track and plus, it is just more fun to have a friend working with you, especially when exercising.

Losing Weight

Okay, now that we have covered motivation, we are now going to cover some basic weight loss tips, tricks and helpful facts.

The first suggestion is to lose your dependency upon fast food; fast food may be convenient but that all that it is good for.

Not only is the food going to be full of grease, but it is chock full of artificial ingredients, fillers and preservatives. None of that is healthy to put in our bodies.

You will need to start doing more cooking and less ordering out of your car window. Now, do not panic, it is possible to put together your own meals without having to spend hours in the kitchen.

Many people do not realize that they can eat healthy and not have to spend a ton of time in the kitchen.

There are times when you will be pressed for time and that you might have to grab a fast bite to eat.

Do not despair because you can still get a healthy meal at a fast food joint or a restaurant and it will still be tasty.

Eating out is the downfall of dieters, unless they know what to order! That is the trick, making smarter menu choices to help you lose weight.

If you are at a restaurant, avoid the foods that are fried, covered in sauce or fatty cuts of meat. Limit your fish intake to once a week, fish tend to absorb toxins from the water that they are in and that will contribute to your man boobs.

Lean proteins such as turkey, chicken, and lean beef are your best choices for at a restaurant. Avoid things that are covered in cheese or sauce, those just add fat and calories.

Ask to keep the sauces taken off and for the cheese to be left off. A tasty and delicious alternative to heavy sauces is to have fresh salsa used instead, this works great with both chicken and lean steak, and it will add flavor and few calories.

Choose to have fruit instead of French fries and always take a pass on the onion rings. Remember that things like potato salad are made with mayonnaise and will be high calorie as well.

Grilled and baked is the best way to order your food, it will be healthier for you, and usually marinated, so that the meat will be flavorful and juicy.

A big mistake people make when they are at a restaurant is that they think a salad is healthy. In a restaurant, the salads often have as many or more calories than the entrees. The reason for that is because the salads usually have so many things added to them, such as egg, cheese, croutons, meats, caramelized nuts or fruits, and salad dressing.

All of those tasty components just adds to the calorie count. The simplest salads are the best to order because they have the least to them and will be healthier, such as a salad with grilled chicken or lean steak and very little else on top.

If you find yourself at a fast food place, ignore the burgers, and go for a veggie burger, a turkey burger or a chicken breast sandwich, grilled, not fried.

Skip the fries and opt for iced tea instead if you get a drink. Instead of a burger joint, go instead of a sandwich place, where you can get a healthy sandwich instead.

Choose lean meats, skip the bacon, and skip the mayonnaise. Mustard has zero calories and it goes with most things, or just use oil and vinegar instead. Opt for whole wheat bread and skip eating white bread totally.

If there is a dish that you are craving, order it. The key to a successful diet is to not deprive yourself of everything that you love, but eat it in moderation and on a limited basis.

So when you eat out, use it as an opportunity to turn one meal into two. Eat half, and take half home! Instant dinner or lunch for another day!

Cut soda from your diet, we already went over this, but it warrants being said again, there is no benefit to drinking soda. Drink something better for you and forget about soda.

You are going to also give up your ice cream, candy, and sweet things. If you have a major sweet tooth that you simply cannot ignore, you can eat in moderation.

Allow yourself a ½ cup of ice cream after dinner nightly and that will be about 120 calories, but do not guess the size of the cup of ice cream, actually measure it out!

Portion control is a big factor. We tend to eat way more than we need to daily, we do so because we can and because we are used to doing so.

Somewhere in our lives, eating too much became a habit and now we must break it.

When you are used to eating a dinner portion that covers your entire plate, and maybe going back for seconds, when you cut your food intake down, you will find that seeing empty plate can be disheartening.

There is a solution to the empty plate blues, buy smaller plates.

Humans are very visual and what we see greatly affects our thinking so if you see a plate that has empty space, where normally there would not be any, your brain will start to think that you are not getting enough food, even though you are.

It will actually work against you because your brain is telling you that there should not be room on your plate and because there is, you must be starving and you will end up overeating.

Smaller plates and bowls is the solution to that. Smaller plates will be the perfect solution for the empty plate blues because you will have that smaller portion, on a smaller plate and no empty space to be seen.

Your brain will not start to think that you are being deprived of food because you will not be seeing empty spaces.

You need to start eating less in order to lose weight. So how can you eat less and still feel full?

There are ways, using smaller plates and bowls is only one-way to do this, there are other tricks to eating less and still feeling full.

Take smaller bites and really chew your food. When you eat fast, you end up overeating and then you get too full.

When you eat slow, it gives your stomach time to tell your brain that you are full and to stop eating. Smaller bites allow you to eat slow and then savor each bite. You will enjoy your meal more and end up eating less.

Spice makes you feel fuller, so add a splash of something spicy to the meal, using fresh salsa with a little bit of kick to it is a great way to give your meal a flavor kick and help you eat less!

Another key to losing weight is to NOT skip a meal that is a big mistake to make. That just tends to make you overeat instead later or that you will eat too much.

Always eat breakfast, even something simple such as some oatmeal or a smoothie is better than eating nothing, or grab some fresh fruit.

The Alkaline Diet

The more acidic your body is, the more out of whack your hormones are, and the more it affects the growth and presence of man boobs.

When you make your body less acidic and more alkaline, it helps to align the hormone balance and thereby reducing your man boobs.

As foods are digested, they become either acidic or alkaline and a sour food, or a food that has acid in it, can actually be alkaline, such as lemon.

Eating a diet high in alkaline foods and low in foods that have an acidic impact on your body is a good way to not only improve your overall health but to help get rid of your man boobs. Your body's PH balance will be more alkaline, which is how you want it to be.

By avoiding the foods that are high acidity foods and eating food that are alkaline and high alkaline, you will be well on your way to getting rid of your man boobs.

It is simple to swap out acidic foods for foods that are more alkaline. Your diet should be 75% alkaline and 25% acidic to give you the balance that you are looking for to optimize your health and the conditions that will help reduce man boobs.

Eat the foods that are listed as acidic and slightly acidic in moderation.

Fruits

Slightly acidic

Canned tomatoes, sweet cherries, blueberries

Moderately alkaline

Banana, apple, acai berry, black currant, tart cherry, blackberries, apricot, dates, coconut, dragon fruit, cranberry, grapefruit, Italian plum, dried fig, gooseberry, grapes, mango, mandarin orange, pomegranate, nectarine, papaya, orange, pineapple, pear, peach, red currant, raspberry, yellow plum, strawberry, rose hips, tangerine, watermelon, tomato

Highly Acidic

Fig, avocado, lime, kiwi, goji berries, lemon

Grains

Acidic

White rice, Bulgar rice, wheat, pasta, corn

Slightly acidic

Barley, basmati rice, brown rice, kamut, oat, spelt

Alkaline

Spelt, quinoa, amaranth, wild rice, buckwheat, barley grass

Legumes

Acidic

Kidney beans, black beans

Slightly acidic

Chickpeas

Slightly alkaline

White beans, lentils, soy beans, lima beans, red beans, mung beans, pinto beans, navy beans

Alkaline

Sprouted beans, soy lecithin, green beans

Vegetables

Acidic

Sauerkraut, canned vegetables, pickled vegetables, frozen vegetables, cooked vegetables (they become acidic when cooked)

Slightly alkaline

Zucchini, basil, watercress, bell peppers, thyme, cauliflower, squash, chives, rhubarb, lamb's lettuce, peas, parsnips, onion

Alkaline

Tomato, artichokes, spinach, bok choy, sorrel, Brussels sprouts, savoy cabbage, cabbage, red cabbage, cayenne pepper, pumpkin, celery, pepper, cilantro, oregano, comfrey, mustard greens, garlic, lettuce, endive

Highly alkaline

Wheat grass, alfalfa, sprouted seeds, broccoli, soy sprouts, cucumber, shave grass, dandelion, **kamu grass**, kale, dog grass

Roots

Slightly alkaline

Potato, carrots, turnip, kohlrabi, yams, rutabaga, white radish, sweet potatoes

Alkaline

Red radish, beets, ginseng

Highly alkaline

Black radish, jicama, ginger

Nuts & Seeds

Acidic

Wheat kernel, peanut butter, chestnuts, peanuts, pecans, pistachios

Slightly acidic

Walnuts, brazil nuts, nutmeg, cashews, macadamia nuts, hazelnut

Slightly alkaline

Sunflower seeds, almonds, pumpkin seeds, raw almond butter, flax seeds, raw pine nuts, sesame seeds, caraway seeds, fennel seeds, cumin seeds

Sugars and Sweeteners

Highly acidic

Sugar, splenda, corn syrup, beet sugar, sweet n low, equal

Acidic

Saccharine, brown rice syrup, sugarcane, chocolate

Slightly acidic

Maple syrup, agave nectar, honey, barley malt syrup

Alkaline

Stevia, blackstrap molasses

Bread

Acidic

White bread, corn tortillas, sourdough bread, pancakes, waffles

Slightly acidic

Spelt bread, rye bread, whole grain bread, sprouted bread, white biscuits, wheat bread

Oils & Fats

Slightly acidic

Sunflower oil, corn oil, canola oil, margarine, cod liver oil

Slightly alkaline

Udo's oil, avocado oil, sesame oil, borage oil, olive oil, coconut oil, marine lipids, flax seed oil, evening primrose oil

Dairy

Acidic

Greek Yogurt, Yogurt, cheese, sour cream, ice cream, egg whites, cream, butter, eggs and egg whites

Slightly acidic

Raw milk, milk, buttermilk

Poultry, Fish & Meat

Highly acidic

Veal, bacon, venison, beef, sausage, buffalo, turkey, canned sardines, pork, lamb, canned tuna, organ meat

Acidic

Tuna, carp, shrimp, chicken, shark, clams, shellfish, cod, sardines, duck, salmon, fresh water fish, scallops, liver, rabbit, lobster, pike, mussels, oysters, ocean fish

Drinks

Acidic

Wine, beer, black tea, processed fruit juice, liquor, sparkling water, coffee, soda

Alkaline

Water, fresh squeezed juice (all natural), green tea, herbal tea

All Other

Highly acidic

Pizza, candy, prescription pills and drugs, cigarettes, chips

Acidic

Mayonnaise, canned foods, soy sauce, breakfast cereals, mustard, microwavable meals and foods, ketchup, popcorn, miso

Slightly acidic

Whey protein powder, hummus, mushrooms, soy protein powder, soymilk, rice milk

Slightly alkaline

Tofu, apple cider vinegar, tempeh, royal jelly, bee pollen

Alkaline

Almond milk, goat milk, baking soda

Therefore, now that you know what foods you should be eating more of, you can begin to plan some meals that are both healthy and will help you get rid of your man boobs.

Get yourself a juicer. With a juicer, you can combine the alkaline foods in any combination that you want to get a great tasting juice and if you want more texture, add some ice to make a smoothie.

Smoothies and juices are a great way to start your day off, they make for a great breakfast and can be made quickly and put in a cup to go so you can enjoy on your way to work.

You can use lettuce leaves to replace tortillas to make tasty wraps, you can combine chopped nuts, vegetables and add spices, using olive oil to mix it all and hold it together and then wrap in the leaf. You will have a tasty and healthy lunch or snack.

Another quick breakfast is to make an omelet with chopped veggies and eggs, leave off the cheese, but you can make a quick and tasty omelet or even just make a veggie and egg scramble. Oatmeal with fruit mixed in is another great breakfast meal.

Soups made from alkaline foods are a great and filling choice, especially on a cold day. The plus side to soups is that you can make them in a big batch, because they store nicely, and then carry only what you want to eat that day to work to heat up.

All you need is a vegetable broth stock and diced vegetables, add some seasonings and simmer until ready! Lentils work nicely as an addition to soups as well. Broccoli soup and vegetable with lentil are soups that make for hearty and filling lunches.

Salads are a great way to eat alkaline foods and you have so many versatile options as to what you want to add for the salads.

You can use different lettuce, remember that the darker leafy lettuces are the best for you, and then add vegetables and alkaline nuts and seeds to give the salad crunch and texture; they work just as well as croutons and are much healthier.

Try mixing olive oil and apple cider vinegar for a salad dressing. Sprinkle some sea salt over the salad for an extra explosion of flavor and lemon, when squeezed over the salad is a tasty flavor addition.

For your dinners, you should have a small portion of a lean protein and then healthy and hearty portions of alkaline vegetables and a salad to go with it.

Use limes and chilies to make sauces with, they will add flavor to the meat; you can use them in olive oil marinades as well.

This healthy diet will get you well on your way towards losing weight, feeling better and getting rid of your unsightly man boobs.

The Stress and Sleep Factors

When you are trying to get rid of your man boobs, sleep is another important factor. Most people do not get enough sleep during the day and they do not even realize it, they just go about their lives thinking that it is normal to not feel well rested but it is not.

Sleeping helps your body help you get rid of your man boobs and even your extra weight.

Avoid foods or beverages with caffeine in them at night, no caffeine after lunch. Sugary foods will also help to keep you awake and nighttime is when your body and mind need to shut down, to rest up and re-charge so try to not snack at least an hour before bed and no caffeine after lunch.

Studies have shown that if you exercise for thirty minutes before going to bed, that you will sleep better. You can go to a gym, use your own gym equipment or even an exercise video, as long as it can gets your heart rate up and you exercise for thirty minutes at a minimum.

When you are done, a hot shower and then bed and you will drift off to sleep much faster than if you had not exercised. Not only does it help you sleep, but it will help you lose that extra weight as well.

Try taking melatonin at night; take it about an hour before bedtime. Melatonin is a natural substance that helps to regulate the bodies sleep cycles and it is non-habit forming, unlike sleeping pills, which are bad for you to take, and very habit forming.

At night, staring at a TV, computer screen, phone, or e-reader device while in bed can actually hinder your ability to sleep.

Your bed is what you sleep in, and if you sit and watch TV, or play on the computer, then when you are in bed, your mind does not equate bed with sleep.

The other devices are usually backlit and that can actually help you stay awake and not help you fall asleep!

Your room at night should be dark, use low-wattage bulbs in the lamps nearest your bed. Reversely, during the day, you need to get as much light exposure as possible, if you are inside, let light into the room by opening the drapes.

By exposing yourself to light during the day and darkness at night, it helps your body stay in the sleep and awake cycle that you want it to.

The other obstacle towards you getting rid of your man boobs is stress. When you are stressed, you release cortisol, which decreases your testosterone, which in turn, contributes to man boobs.

The more stress you are under and the longer you are stressed, the worse you man boobs will get.

Stress also causes a variety of health problems, so you need to get a handle on your stress if you want to be healthy and get rid of, and keep your man boobs gone.

The chapter on the importance of breathing has a great breathing exercise that you should do at least three times during the day and again whenever you are feeling stressed.

The best thing about the deep breathing exercise is that you can do it anywhere and instantly feel better.

If there is a situation that is causing stress in your life, take steps to solve it. Ignoring a situation is unhealthy, especially when with communication; most problems can be worked out.

If there is a stressful situation that you can avoid, such as traffic, do so! If you hate traffic, then leave for work a half hour earlier than normal, and then read your paper or grab a healthy breakfast someplace near the office.

If a certain person causes stress, do your best to avoid them. If you cannot avoid stress, then do your best to manage it.

If you are stressed over a situation that you cannot control, accept that you cannot control it and you will have less stress.

There is no point in worrying about things that you have no ability to control; the outcome will be the same whether or not you stress about it, so why put yourself through that?

Stop taking on so much responsibility. If you have something that can be delegated, do so. Nobody says that you have to be superman, delegate.

No one person can handle everything so stop trying. Taking on more than you can handle is a common cause of stress.

Meditation is a great way to relieve stress. You can do so at home, before bed. You can buy guided meditation cds and DVDs or you can find one on YouTube. A guided meditation will help you clear your mind and allow it to quiet down for bed.

Exercises to Get Rid of Man Boobs

Changing what you eat alone will not help, especially if you are overweight. You need to exercise as well, not only to lose weight as a whole, but exercises that target your man boobs specifically.

We will go over both general and targeted exercises in this chapter, because both are important, more so if you are already overweight.

We are going to start with some easy tips for working some extra exercise into your day, these will be especially good for those of you who are busy, or not very active.

Believe it or not, several small changes made to your daily routine can add up to having a big impact on your weight loss.

When you get to work, you tend to park up front, as close as you can, right? If the weather is good, park as far away as you can and walk, if you are in a parking garage; take the stairs, the extra bit of walking ads up quickly!

Inside the building, use the elevator instead of stairs and you will be amazed at how much difference that little bit of extra walking each day will bring you.

Cardio

Cardio workouts are great for weight loss and for helping to lose your man boobs. Not only will cardio help you lose weight but also it helps to keep your heart healthy and will give you stamina and endurance.

Cardio is also a great stress reliever and helps your lungs get stronger at the same time.

You should get at least thirty minutes of cardio exercise for a minimum of three days a week and a maximum of five days out of the week.

Do not do your cardio at the same time that you do your resistance training; they should be spaced out by several hours.

If you have the money for a class, martial arts are a great cardio workout. Not only will you learn something fun, but you will also have a fun workout while learning discipline, breathing, and the principles of martial arts.

Swimming is a great cardio exercise, as long as you have access to a pool. If you do, swimming is a good way to tone, burn fat and shed those extra pounds, along with your man boobs.

The front crawl and the butterfly are two strokes that rely on the pectoral muscles and will be good for weight loss and reducing the size of your man boobs.

Walking is a cardio exercise that anybody can do. Even if you are obese, you can walk, you do not have to set any records for speed or distance, you just need to get moving.

You can buy a treadmill, use one at the gym, or just go for a good, old-fashioned walk outside!

Bring water that is infused with lemon with you and go enjoy a nice walk. Use a pedometer to see how many steps you take and you will be surprised!

The more you walk, the more you will see that you can walk further and faster without running out of breath.

You will begin to look and feel better and there is not better ego boost than being able to easily do a walk route that once had you panting and wanting to drop! Once you get used to walking, you can begin to jog or even run.

If you own a bike, you can begin taking long bike rides as your cardio. Instead of a slow ride, you push yourself so that your heart rate increases slightly. If you do not break a sweat, it is not cardio!

An elliptical machine is great cardio because not only are you working hard at it, but also it engages your arms and chest muscles as well, making it a full body cardio workout, it is very effective.

Step machines, stationary bikes, and rowing machines are also very good choices, especially rowing machines because they will engage the chest muscles.

If you enjoy sports, that could be your cardio activity right there. Football, basketball, soccer, tennis, and racquetball are all cardio sports.

You can find an amateur league and join up or play with friends or at the gym. You can buy a jump rope and do thirty minutes of jump rope as your cardio or even jumping jacks.

Strength and resistance training

The easiest and most basic way to work the area of your chest is to do push-ups daily. Push-ups are easy; they work with your own body weight and are excellent for targeting your pectorals, as well as your arms.

A basic push-up is simple, with your toes and your palms on the floor have your legs straight and then slowly lower yourself to the floor, keeping your body straight and even.

Just as your nose nearly touches the floor, reverse and push yourself back to the original position. Try to do one set of 10 to begin with and then increase it to two sets of ten, then three sets of ten, then one set of 15, then two sets of 15, etc.

For this next exercise you need a wall that is clear of furniture, you can do this in the hallway or the entryway, anywhere that you have access to a section of the wall where you will not be knocking anything over.

Stand with your back to the wall and then lower yourself so that you are "sitting" against the wall, hold in this sitting position for thirty seconds and then stand up.

Repeat this ten times.

Regular sit-ups also do the job. Lie on your back, put your hands behind your head and raise your knees up in the air and then sit up and try touch your right elbow to your left knee as you raise up, this means that you have to tilt your elbow to connect, and that is fine, just keep your hands behind your head and then go back to the starting position and then repeat, using the other elbow and knee.

Keep repeating this, start off with a set of 15 and then build up like with the push-ups.

If you have access to weight machines, you want to use machines that target your chest muscles. However, you can use free weights to lose man boobs, so you should invest in a set of barbells for your home, or use the ones at the gym; a weight bench will also be a good investment, because you will need to keep up the routines after the man boobs are gone in order to keep them off.

Should I Get Surgery?

For persistent man boobs, the question always arises, should I get surgery? There is no clear-cut answer to this, but our position is that surgery should always be a last resort.

If you are overweight, and your man boobs are simply fat deposits, then they can do liposuction, which is painful, expensive and can leave scarring.

In addition, there is a risk of infection and of having a doctor who is not qualified. If you look into this and they give you a price that is too good to be true, it very likely is and you should walk away.

This procedure is usually done just under your areola or under your arm, the surgeon will cut open and then go through that opening to remove extra fat and glandular tissue, drains will be put in and then the surgery will be over.

However, if your man boobs are due to enlarged mammary glands and tissue, surgery is an option. A surgeon will have to cut away and remove the excess glandular tissue.

For men where nothing else worked, this is the last resort. Keep in mind, if you are overweight, then you will still have unhealthy fat on your body, and it will migrate back up to your chest. You should only consider surgery if you are already fit and healthy.

Also, if you have the surgery but continue to have all of the same habits that you had before, such as eating and drinking the same foods that cause the hormonal imbalance to begin with, your problem will only end up coming back.

Surgery is a painful and expensive thing and you do not want to endure it twice.

You will, of course, have to be screened for any medical conditions that could be causing your man boobs, but you already should have gotten those checked out.

In the first chapter we discussed what some of the medical reasons for this condition are and that you should be seen by a doctor. If you have not, you will get screened prior to surgery.

As with any surgery, there are risks. Risks include infection, bleeding, scars, uneven breasts, fluid retention, and fluid loss.

No matter which kind of surgery, you will have a scar or scars. Will the scars cause you as much concern as the man boobs did? If the answer is yes, then you should not get the surgery.

Conclusion

Man boobs are a common concern with men of all ages. Often, they show at adolescence and then go away with puberty or shortly thereafter. Sometimes, it does not go away and sometimes, there is no problem until later on in life and then you develop man boobs.

If you have man boobs, always get a full physical from your doctor. There are a variety of health issues that can cause this and as with any health issue, the earlier it is caught, the easier it is to cure.

Some of the conditions can be very serious, such as breast cancer. Men are not immune to breast cancer but many do not believe that it can happen to them, but it can.

Whenever your body is doing something that it did not used to do, such as develop breasts, you need to see a doctor.

If your doctor tells you that you have no medical reasons and that you are either overweight or have a hormone imbalance, or a combination of the two, then you are not stuck living with your man boobs.

You can control your environment to limit the toxins that end up in your body, causing that hormonal imbalance.

Make the switch to all natural cleaners, limit the plastic that your food comes into contact with and drink filtered water are all a good way to start.

Keeping your body in an alkaline state is another way to help your hormones balance.

By using our chart of what foods are acidic and to be avoided and what foods are alkaline and should be eaten, you can make healthy and smart eating choices that will begin to reduce your man boobs.

You need to stay hydrated, get enough sleep, learn to breathe deeply and steadily and get rid of your extra stress as well.

It can be hard to stop eating the foods that you are used to eating, but it is for your health and once you stop eating them, you will begin to feel so much better that you will wonder why you ever ate them to begin with!

Losing weight is another thing that must be done. If you are overweight, your man boobs will persist.

Getting yourself healthy is the only way for you to get rid of your man boobs once and for all.

Cardio and strength training is the best way to shed your unwanted pounds and your man boobs, and if you cannot afford a gym, you can always do laps around the block while carrying weights, or even just walking without them.

The point is, there are many things that you can do to reduce and get rid of your man boobs, and you just have to be willing to make the changes.

Once you begin to make the changes and you can see the difference, you will wonder why you waited so long. The body that you have always wanted is waiting for you, get started now!

www.ingramcontent.com/pod-product-compliance
Lightning Source LLC
Chambersburg PA
CBHW020355290526
45785CB00005B/2302